THE 10-DAY DETOX

THE 10-DAY DETOX

Cleanse Your Body, Clear Your Mind

TRISTAN EVERGREEN

QuantumQuill Press

CONTENTS

Copyright © 2024 by Tristan Evergreen

All rights reserved. No part of this book may be reproduced in any manner whatsoever without written permission except in the case of brief quotations embodied in critical articles and reviews.

First Printing, 2024

Introduction to The 10-Day Detox: Cleanse Your Body, Clear Your Mind

Welcome to an extraordinary excursion that will direct you through a far reaching detoxification process, planned not exclusively to scrub your body yet additionally to clear your brain. This excursion is about something beyond eliminating poisons from your eating regimen; it's tied in with resetting your general existence, cultivating a freshly discovered feeling of imperativeness, and making ready for a better way of life.

The Pith of Detoxification

In our cutting edge world, we are presented to a horde of poisons everyday. From the air we inhale to the food we devour, our bodies ingest different substances that can influence our wellbeing. While the body is normally outfitted with frameworks to take out these poisons, the over-burden can be overpowering, prompting a scope of medical problems, from exhaustion and cerebrum haze to stomach related issues and persistent diseases.

Detoxification, hence, turns into a crucial cycle to help our body's inherent capacity to purge itself. It's a purposeful delay we take, a cognizant decision to diminish the weight on our detoxification organs and frameworks. This 10-day detox program is intended to launch that interaction, giving your body the break it necessities to effectively eliminate these poisons, restore, and fix.

The Objectives of The 10-Day Detox

This program is worked around the center objective of reviving your body and psyche. Over the course of the following 10 days, you will leave on an excursion to:

•Take out destructive poisons from your eating routine and climate, giving your body a more clear way to mend and restore.

•Help your actual wellbeing, through painstakingly chosen food sources and enhancements that help detoxification, close by proactive tasks that animate your body's regular detox processes.

•Improve mental lucidity and close to home prosperity, with rehearses intended to lessen pressure, clear your brain, and develop a feeling of internal harmony.

•Establish the groundwork for reasonable way of life changes, outfitting you with the information and propensities to keep supporting your wellbeing past these 10 days.

What's in store

The 10-Day Detox program is organized at this point adaptable, recognizing that every individual's body and detox needs are extraordinary. This is the thing you can anticipate from the program:

1. Guided Day to day Plans: Every day of the detox will be framed for you, including what to eat, discretionary enhancements to help your detox process, proactive tasks, and care rehearses.

2. Nutritional Help: You'll be acquainted with an eating routine wealthy in entire, supplement thick food sources, intended to help your body's detoxification frameworks. The program incorporates detox-accommodating recipes and test dinner intends to make the cycle as smooth and pleasant as could really be expected.

3. Physical Exercises: Delicate yet compelling activities will be prescribed to supplement the detox cycle, improving course and advancing the end of poisons through sweat.

4. Mindfulness and Emotional well-being Practices: Procedures like reflection, journaling, and breathing activities will be consolidated to assist with clearing your brain and lessen pressure, which is fundamental for a fruitful detox.

Getting ready for Your Excursion

As we leave on this detox venture, it's vital to plan both intellectually and truly. This implies laying out reasonable objectives, establishing a steady climate, and maybe in particular, moving toward the cycle with a receptive outlook and a guarantee to taking care of oneself.

Keep in mind, detoxification isn't just about the actual expulsion of poisons; it's additionally about making space for new, better propensities and viewpoints. This program is a potential chance to stop, reflect, and deliberately pick a way toward better wellbeing and prosperity.

We should Start

As you stand at the edge of this 10-day venture, recollect that you're not simply setting out on a momentary detox program; you're venturing out toward a more dynamic, solid, and careful approach to everyday life. This guide is here to help you constantly, offering itemized directions, consolation, and the devices you want to succeed.

Thus, take a full breath, and we should step forward into this excursion together, with the common objective of purifying your body and clearing your psyche. Welcome to The 10-Day Detox.

Understanding Detoxification

The Investigation of Detoxification

Detoxification is a foremost natural connection, where the body methodicallly perceives, kills, and takes out hazardous substances. These substances can be both endogenous, beginning from inside the body, as metabolic wastes, and exogenous, coming from external sources like toxins, pesticides, and took care of food added substances.

At the focal point of the body's detoxification structure are the liver, kidneys, stomach related organs, lungs, lymphatic system, and skin. Each organ expects an essential part:

•Liver: The liver channels and kills harms, setting them up for safe end.

•Kidneys: The kidneys wipe out aftereffects from the blood and release them in pee.

•Stomach related organs: The gastrointestinal part discards harms through the fertilizer and hinders reabsorption into the circulatory framework.

•Lungs: The lungs expel temperamental substances through exhalation.

•Lymphatic Structure: This association exhausts and channels lymph fluid, killing waste and toxins.

•Skin: The skin releases harms through sweat and fills in as a limit against outside poisons.

The capability of these systems is fundamental for staying aware of prosperity. In any case, in our contemporary environment, the body's detox cutoff can be overwhelmed due to the extraordinary volume and combination of toxins we're introduced to regular. This over-weight can provoke an improvement of toxic substances in our tissues, potentially causing an extent of clinical issues.

What Harms Mean for the Body and Cerebrum

Toxic substances can influence basically every system in the body, provoking a variety of clinical issues. Presumably the most notable effects include:

•Stomach related Issues: Toxic substances can disturb the stomach microbiome, inciting enlarging, stoppage, and other stomach related issues.

•Depletion: Hoarding of toxic substances can impact mitochondrial capacity, diminishing energy creation.

•Mental Ability: Toxic substances can cross the blood-frontal cortex deterrent, conceivably provoking brain fog, mental deterioration, and reduced mental capacity.

•Insusceptible System Disguise: Tenacious receptiveness to toxins can overburden the safe structure, making the body more vulnerable to pollutions and diseases.

•Hormonal Disproportionate qualities: Various toxins can impersonate synthetics, disturbing endocrine capacity and provoking an extent of hormonal issues.

The mental and up close and personal impacts of toxin receptiveness are comparatively basic. Stress, pressure, and mental episodes can be exacerbated by the physiological effects of toxins, creating a cycle that can be attempting to break without intercession.

Benefits of Detoxing

Leaving on a detox program offers different benefits, including:

•Updated Energy Levels: By taking out harms and improving mitochondrial ability, detoxing can in a general sense help energy levels.

•Further created Absorption: Detoxification maintains stomach prosperity, inciting better enhancement ingestion and end of waste.

•All the more clear Skin: As the skin clears harms, you could see overhauls in shading and by and large prosperity.

•Weight decrease: Detoxing can help with reseting the body's assimilation, supporting weight decrease and the abatement of muscle versus fat.

•Mental Clarity: Diminishing toxin weight can incite unrivaled mental capacities, similar to fixation and memory.

•Significant Thriving: By keeping an eye on the real pieces of prosperity, detoxing can similarly incite better close than home balance and stress the leaders.

The Exhaustive Method for managing Detoxification

A compelling detox program isn't just about what you wipe out from your body and life; it's in like manner about what you add. Merging enhancement thick food assortments, partaking in dynamic work, and practicing care are major pieces of an extensive detox plan. This approach maintains the body's typical detoxification processes as well as advances a lifestyle that constantly supports physical and mental health.

Detoxification is an outing that requires liability and care. Sorting out the science behind it, the effects of toxins on the body and mind, and the clear benefits of detoxing sets areas of strength for a point for this momentous experience. As we push ahead, we'll guide you through making arrangements for your detox, outfitting you with the instruments and data to investigate this trip really.

Pre-Detox Preparation

Prior to leaving on your 10-day detox venture, it's pivotal to plan both intellectually and truly. This readiness guarantees you can boost the advantages of your detox, making way for an effective purge. Here, we'll dive into systems for mental planning, actual status, and establishing a strong climate for your detox process.

Mental Readiness: Developing the Right Outlook

Grasping Your 'Why': Start by pondering your purposes behind endeavor this detox. Whether it's to work on your wellbeing, acquire energy, or just to challenge yourself, having an unmistakable comprehension of your 'why' will keep you roused all through the excursion.

Setting Practical Assumptions: While detoxing can bring critical medical advantages, setting sensible expectations is significant. Recognize that there might be testing days, yet recollect that these are ventures toward a more noteworthy objective.

Embracing Change: Free yourself up to the progressions that will come, both during and after the detox. This transparency can make the interaction smoother and really fulfilling.

Actual Planning: Preparing Your Body

Slow Decrease of Poisons: In the days paving the way to your detox, begin lessening the admission of handled food varieties, caffeine, sugar, and liquor. This continuous decrease can assist with limiting withdrawal side effects and make the progress simpler.

Hydration: Expanding your water admission prior to beginning the detox assists with starting the most common way of flushing out poisons. Go for the gold 8 glasses of water a day.

Healthful Help: Begin integrating more detox-accommodating food varieties into your eating routine, like mixed greens, natural products, and entire grains. These food varieties give fundamental supplements and fiber, supporting the detox interaction.

Active work: In the event that you're not currently in a standard work-out everyday practice, start presenting light proactive tasks like strolling or yoga. This will help launch your body's regular detoxification processes.

Establishing a Strong Climate

Loading Up: Guarantee you have every one of the fundamental fixings and supplies for your detox, including any suggested supplements. Having all that available will make it more straightforward to stay on course.

Coordinating Your Space: Make a spotless, coordinated living space that upholds your detox objectives. This could mean cleaning up your kitchen, setting up a peaceful space for reflection, or setting up your exercise region.

Looking for Help: Educate loved ones regarding your detox plans and, if conceivable, search out a detox pal. Having backing can give extra inspiration and responsibility.

Advanced Detox: Consider lessening screen time and computerized interruptions. This can assist with bringing down feelings of anxiety and further develop rest quality, the two of which are valuable for your detox process.

Planning for the Close to home Excursion

Detoxing isn't simply an actual cycle; it's a personal one too. The progressions your body goes through can influence your state of mind and feelings. Getting ready for this part of the detox is similarly just about as significant as the actual arrangement.

Journaling: Begin a detox diary to report your excursion, including your sentiments, difficulties, and victories. This can be a significant device for reflection and inspiration.

Care Practices: Start rehearsing care or contemplation to assist with overseeing pressure and feelings. Indeed, even a couple of moments daily can have a tremendous effect.

Taking care of oneself Ceremonies: Plan to consolidate taking care of oneself exercises that you appreciate, like showers, perusing, or investing energy in nature. These can assist with supporting your profound prosperity during the detox.

The Last Days Before Your Detox

Over the most recent couple of days prior to beginning your detox, center around setting your aims for the excursion ahead. Survey your objectives, the arrangement for every day, and how you'll oversee likely difficulties. This is likewise a great opportunity to progressively begin executing the day to day schedules you'll follow during the detox, like dinner timings and work-out schedules.

Rest and Unwinding: Guarantee you're getting satisfactory rest and permitting time for unwinding. A very much refreshed body and psyche are stronger and prepared for the detox cycle.

Last Check: Go through your agenda one final opportunity to guarantee everything is set up for Day 1. This incorporates food, supplements, and any devices you'll require for exercise and unwinding rehearses.

Embracing the Excursion

As you stand on the edge of your 10-day detox, recall that this excursion is about something beyond the physical purge. It's a valuable chance to reset propensities, to listen profoundly to your body, and to support a more careful relationship with food and wellbeing.

Move toward every day of the detox with interest and empathy for yourself. There will be ups and downs, however each step is a piece of the groundbreaking system. By getting ready completely and embracing the excursion ahead, you're getting yourself positioned for a fruitful and significant detox insight.

CHAPTER 1

Day 1: Setting the Foundation

Wake-up routine

Hydration: Begin your day with a glass of warm lemon water. This basic ceremony helps with assimilation and launches the liver's detoxification cycle.

Care Practice: Participate in a 10-minute reflection zeroing in on your breath. This training helps focus your considerations and set a positive expectation for the afternoon.

Breakfast

Detox Smoothie: Mix a combination of spinach, frozen blueberries, a portion of a banana, chia seeds, and almond milk. This supplement thick smoothie assists with stimulating your body and backing detoxification.

Supplemental Help

Multivitamin: Take a far reaching multivitamin to guarantee you're getting fundamental supplements that help by and large detox pathways.

Actual work

Morning Walk: A 30-minute lively stroll in nature. This delicate activity upholds lymphatic flow and lifts temperament.

Early in the day

Nibble: A little modest bunch of crude almonds and an apple. This tidbit gives fiber and sound fats to keep you satisfied.

Lunch

Quinoa Salad: Set up a serving of mixed greens with cooked quinoa, blended greens, cucumber, avocado, and a lemon-tahini dressing. This feast is wealthy in fiber and solid fats, helping with detoxification and energy upkeep.

Evening Custom

Hydration Lift: Drink some green tea. Its cell reinforcements support liver capability and give a delicate jolt of energy.

Care Break: Require 5 minutes for profound breathing activities to assist with decreasing pressure and pull together your energy.

Actual work

Yoga: Take part in a 20-minute delicate yoga meeting zeroing in on detoxifying presents, for example, turns that animate processing and dissemination.

Supper

Steamed Vegetables and Lentils: A light, supporting feast comprising of steamed broccoli, carrots, and lentils, prepared with spices and a dash of olive oil. This blend upholds detoxification while being delicate on the stomach related framework.

Evening Custom

Appreciation Journaling: Endure 10 minutes writing in your diary, zeroing in on appreciation. Think about the positive parts of your day and the means you've taken on your detox process.

Groundwork for Rest: Participate in a loosening up action, for example, perusing or washing up with Epsom salts, to advance a peaceful night's rest.

Reflection

End Day 1 by pondering your encounters, difficulties, and victories. Note any sentiments or responses in your detox diary. This reflection assists with expanding care and mindfulness all through the detox interaction.

CHAPTER 2

Day 2: Deepening the Detox Process

As you enter Day 2 of your detox process, your body starts to conform to the changes. The present spotlight is on improving detoxification while guaranteeing you feel sustained and upheld.

Wake-up routine

Awaken Drink: Begin with a glass of warm water mixed with a cut of new ginger. Ginger is famous for its mitigating properties and can assist with animating absorption.

Care Practice: Take part in a 10-minute yoga meeting zeroed in on delicate extending and relaxing. Yoga postures, for example, turns can assist with invigorating assimilation and backing the body's regular detoxification processes.

Breakfast

Avocado Toast on Sans gluten Bread: Pound a portion of an avocado on a cut of toasted without gluten bread, finished off with a sprinkle of hemp seeds and a shower of olive oil. Avocado gives solid fats and fiber, while hemp seeds add a protein help.

Early in the day

Green Juice: Set up a green juice with kale, celery, green apple, lemon, and a piece of ginger. This invigorating juice gives an extra portion of supplements and compounds to help detoxification.

Active work: Participate quickly of moderate high-impact work out. An energetic walk or a delicate bicycle ride can expand your pulse and dissemination, improving the detox interaction.

Lunch

Lentil Soup with Salad Greens: Partake in a bowl of natively constructed or locally acquired lentil soup, guaranteeing it's low in sodium and liberated from added substances. Add a small bunch of spinach or kale for an additional supplement support. Lentils are an extraordinary wellspring of protein and fiber, helping with processing and poison disposal.

Evening

Hydration Update: Proceed with your admission of water, holding back nothing 8 glasses over the course of the day. Consider adding cuts of cucumber or berries to your water for added flavor and supplements.

Careful Second: Require 5-10 minutes for a directed reflection zeroing in on detoxification and recharging. Perception can be a useful asset in supporting the body's detox endeavors.

Supper

Heated Yam with a Side of Barbecued Asparagus: A prepared yam is wealthy in fiber and beta-carotene, a cell reinforcement that upholds liver wellbeing. Go with it with barbecued asparagus, which is known for its diuretic properties, assisting with flushing out poisons.

Evening Custom

Natural Tea: Taste on some milk thorn tea. Milk thorn is known for its liver-defensive impacts and can help with the detoxification cycle.

Intelligent Journaling: Consider the day, zeroing in on any physical or profound changes you've taken note. Recognize any troubles and commend the achievements of the day.

Groundwork for Day 3: Look forward to Day 3's arrangement. Set up any food sources or put away opportunity for exercises you've arranged, changing in view of your encounters today.

Day 2 Recap and Reflection

Finishing Day 2, you could begin to see unpretentious changes in your energy levels or absorption as your body keeps on adjusting to the detox program. It's critical to pay attention to your body and change depending on the situation, guaranteeing you're furnishing it with enough sustenance and rest. Keep in mind, detoxification isn't just about end yet in addition about recharging and recuperating.

CHAPTER 3

Day 3: Nurturing Your Body and Soul

Entering Day 3, you could start to feel the detox cycle all the more significantly. It's daily to support both your body and soul, zeroing in on food sources and exercises that recharge and reestablish.

Wake-up routine

Awaken Drink: Polish off a glass of warm water with a teaspoon of apple juice vinegar. This tonic can assist with adjusting your body's pH levels and animate stomach related compounds.

Care Practice: Endure 10 minutes rehearsing appreciation contemplation. Center around the parts of your life you're appreciative for, which can emphatically impact your psychological and close to home state, supporting the detox cycle.

Breakfast

Berry and Almond Spread Smoothie: Mix some blended berries (strawberries, blueberries, raspberries) with a tablespoon of almond margarine, a modest bunch of spinach, and almond milk. Berries are high in cancer prevention agents, and almond spread gives sound fats and protein to supported energy.

Early in the day

Natural Coffee Break: Partake in some home grown tea like peppermint or chamomile. These spices can help processing and affect the psyche and body.

Active work: Practice 15 minutes of Qigong or delicate extending works out. These practices can assist with animating energy stream (Qi) in the body and upgrade detoxification.

Lunch

Kale and Avocado Plate of mixed greens with Lemon Dressing: Prepare a serving of mixed greens with crude kale, cuts of avocado, cherry tomatoes, and cucumber. Dress with lemon juice, olive oil, and a sprinkle of ocean salt. This salad is loaded with fiber, sound fats, and nutrients to help detoxification and energy levels.

Evening

Hydration Update: Keep up your water consumption, holding back nothing hydration objective. Adding new mint or a press of lime can give assortment and extra stomach related benefits.

Careful Second: Step outside for a concise stroll in nature or put shortly in a green space. Interfacing with nature can assist with lessening pressure and work on your mind-set.

Supper

Barbecued Lemon and Spice Chicken with Steamed Vegetables: Set up a lean chicken bosom marinated in lemon juice, olive oil, and spices. Present with a side of steamed broccoli and carrots. This dinner gives top notch protein and cancer prevention agents without overpowering the stomach related framework.

Evening Custom

Foot Splash: Set up a warm foot drench with Epsom salts and a couple of drops of rejuvenating balm like lavender or eucalyptus. Splashing your feet can assist with loosening up the body and further develop rest quality.

Intelligent Journaling: Consider your encounters and sentiments from Day 3. Seeing any themes or changes in your physical or profound state can give bits of knowledge into your detox process.

Groundwork for Day 4: Audit the exercises and dinners made arrangements for Day 4. Planning ahead of time can assist with guaranteeing a smooth continuation of your detox program.

Day 3 Recap and Reflection

Toward the finish of Day 3, you're profoundly submerged in the detox cycle. It's a critical time when your body changes and possibly starts to give more recognizable indications of detoxification, like expanded energy or clearness of psyche. Embrace these changes, realizing each step in the right direction is a stage toward worked on prosperity.

CHAPTER 4

Day 4: Strengthening Detox Pathways

By Day 4, your body is changing according to the detox plan. Today, we'll focus in on building up your body's detox pathways, organizing further refining rehearses with managing food sources to help your plan's customary cycles.

Mix plan

Blend Drink: Begin with a glass of warm water infused with new cuts of turmeric and a spot of weak pepper. Turmeric contains curcumin, a compound strong regions for with and cell support properties, while faint pepper revives its ingestion.

Care Practice: Participate in a 15-minute breathing improvement focused in on basic, stomach relaxing. This kind of breathing can help with fortifying the lymphatic structure, an essential piece of your body's detoxification part.

Breakfast

Grain with Flaxseeds and Berries: Set up a bowl of oats using water or almond milk. Top with ground flaxseeds, a little pack of berries, and a sprinkle of pure maple syrup. Oats are high in beta-glucans, dissolvable fibers that help with controlling glucose and sponsorship upkeep, while flaxseeds are wealthy in omega-3 unsaturated fats and lignans that advance hormonal understanding and detoxification.

Rapidly in the day

Green Juice: Make a juice with cucumber, parsley, green apple, lemon, and a handle of ginger. This restoring grant is stacked with chlorophyll, improvements, and minerals, supporting cleansing the blood and supporting liver cutoff.

Dynamic work: Require a 30-minute fiery walk or participate in another sort of moderate cardiovascular movement to assist dispersal and sponsorship with perspiring, another detoxification course.

Lunch

Broccoli and Chickpea Salad: Get steamed broccoli alongside cooked chickpeas, diced red onion, and a tahini-lemon dressing. Broccoli is a cruciferous vegetable that contains sulforaphane, a compound that stays aware of the liver's detoxification motivations, while chickpeas give fiber and protein.

Evening

Hydration Update: Continue to hydrate throughout the span of the day. Consider embedding your water with cuts of lemon and cucumber for extra detoxifying benefits and flavor.

Cautious Second: Convey time for a short, coordinated shrewdness focused in on recovering and cleaning. Envisioning your body conveying harms and fascinating enhancements can stay aware of the detox relationship on a psychological level.

Dinner

Warmed Cod with a Side of Quinoa and Asparagus: Partake in a piece of coordinated cod ready with flavors and lemon, served nearby quinoa and steamed asparagus. Cod gives lean protein and omega-3 unsaturated fats, while quinoa offers a complete protein profile and asparagus assists with kidney detoxification.

Evening Custom

Detox Tea: Taste on some detox tea containing flavors like milk thistle, dandelion, or vex. These flavors support liver and kidney limit, fundamental organs in the detoxification cycle.

Clever Journaling: Slice out an opportunity to journal about your day. How are you feeling, in actuality and mentally? See any burdens and recognition your victories, paying little respect to how little.

Foundation for Day 5: Anticipate Day 5, dissecting your banquet plan and booked works out. Setting up your suppers early and figuring out your day can help with staying aware of energy in your detox cycle.

Day 4 Recap and Reflection

As you wrap up Day 4, you could start to see more imparted effects of the detox. Focusing in on your body during this time and change your activities and diet dependent upon the situation is fundamental. The practices agreeable today point with assistance and further encourage your body's normal detoxification pathways, progressing in customary achievement and prospering.

Day 5: Embracing Renewal and Replenishment

Arriving at Day 5 denotes the midpoint of your detox process. The present spotlight is on recharging and renewal, incorporating food varieties and exercises that support your body and improve your feeling of prosperity.

Wake-up routine

Awaken Drink: Partake in a glass of water with new mint and a cut of lime. This mix is reviving and serves to launch processing with a delicate arousing for your faculties.

Care Practice: Practice a 10-minute meeting of delicate yoga or extending, zeroing in on represents that open and prolong the body. This actual receptiveness can reflect an inward receptiveness to the detoxification and reestablishment processes.

Breakfast

Chia Seed Pudding with Kiwi and Coconut: Douse chia seeds in almond milk for the time being, and top with cut kiwi and a sprinkle of destroyed coconut in the first part of the day. Chia seeds are stacked with fiber, omega-3 unsaturated fats, and protein, making this a filling and nutritious beginning to your day.

Early in the day

Home grown Coffee Break: Pick a natural tea that you see as consoling or fortifying, like rosehip or ginger tea. The two choices offer medical advantages, including L-ascorbic acid and mitigating properties.

Active work: Participate in a low-power Pilates exercise for 20-30 minutes. Pilates can assist with working on your adaptability and center strength while advancing detoxification through lymphatic waste and expanded flow.

Lunch

Spinach and Quinoa Stuffed Ringer Peppers: Burrow out chime peppers and fill them with a combination of cooked quinoa, spinach, onions, and flavors, then, at that point, prepare. This feast is dynamic, loaded with supplements, and supports supported energy levels.

Evening

Hydration Update: Keep on focusing on hydration, expecting to consume liquids consistently over the course of the day. Adding new spices or a sprinkle of natural product juice to your water can give assortment and extra supplements.

Careful Second: Dispense a couple of moments for profound breathing activities, zeroing in on breathing out completely to support setting poisons free from the body and brain.

Supper

Simmered Turmeric Cauliflower with Lentils: Serve broiled cauliflower prepared with turmeric and dark pepper close by a part of cooked lentils. This feast isn't just delightful yet in addition loaded with calming advantages and fundamental supplements to help detoxification.

Evening Custom

Loosening up Shower: Draw a shower with lavender or chamomile natural oil and Epsom salts. The warm water assists with loosening up muscles, while the Epsom salts help in drawing out poisons.

Intelligent Journaling: Invest some energy considering your detox process up to this point. Note any progressions you've seen in your physical, profound, or mental state, and consider what practices or food varieties have had the main effect.

Groundwork for Day 6: Review the arrangement for Day 6, guaranteeing you have regardless of fundamental fixings and setting time for planned exercises. Change in light of your encounters and how your body is answering the detox.

Day 5 Recap and Reflection

Partially through the detox, this is a critical second to perceive the headway you've made and to recalibrate if essential. The present accentuation on restoration and recharging is intended to feed your body profoundly and encourage a feeling of revival. As you push ahead, keep on paying attention to your body's signals and change your detox intend to suit your developing requirements.

CHAPTER 6

Day 6: Intensifying Detoxification Efforts

On Day 6, you've crossed the midpoint and are as of now diving further into the detox collaboration. The current plan is expected to uplift detoxification attempts with an accentuation on supporting liver ability, growing finish of toxic substances, and supporting the body with significantly purging food sources and activities.

Awaken schedule

Stir Drink: Taste on a blend of warm water, lemon juice, and a touch of cayenne pepper. This hot start fortifies retention, helps processing, and supports liver detoxification.

Care Practice: Begin the day with a 15-minute examination focusing in on cleansing and reclamation. Picture your body conveying toxins and imagine yourself stacking up with vigorous, recovering energy.

Breakfast

Detox Green Smoothie: Blend spinach, kale, a little green apple, a part of a cucumber, a tablespoon of ground flaxseed, and a squash of lemon juice with water. This supplement rich smoothie maintains detoxification and gives an upheld shock of energy.

Promptly in the day

Local Short breather: Participate in some regular tea, for instance, burdock root or vex leaf. These flavors are known for their blood-purifying and diuretic properties, assisting with the removal of toxic substances.

Dynamic work: Participate in a 30-minute gathering of cardiovascular movement, such as running, swimming, or cycling. Growing your heartbeat helps with additional creating blood stream and advances sweating, a trademark detoxification process.

Lunch

Arugula and Beet Salad with Walnuts: Join arugula, cut cooked beets, walnuts, and a fundamental olive oil and squeezed apple vinegar dressing. Beets support liver prosperity and detoxification, while walnuts give omega-3 unsaturated fats and arugula is affluent in cell fortifications.

Evening

Hydration Update: Remain mindful of your water utilization, pulling out all the stops 8-10 glasses throughout the span of the day. Infuse your water with cuts of citrus regular items or flavors like mint to redesign its detoxifying properties.

Cautious Second: Have a break for a fragile broadening meeting, focusing in on improvements that stimulate the stomach locale to help handling and detoxification.

Dinner

Lemon Garlic Warmed Salmon with a Side of Steamed Broccoli: Set up a salmon filet with a marinade of lemon juice, garlic, and flavors, and plan. Present with steamed broccoli, which contains increases that help the body's detoxification synthetics.

Evening Custom

Dry Brushing: Before your night shower, practice dry brushing using a trademark fiber brush. Start from your feet and move upwards in extensive, smooth strokes toward your heart. This preparing quickens the lymphatic system, assisting with the ejection of toxins.

Shrewd Journaling: Consider your progression and how you're feeling at this more significant period of the detox. Note any physical, mental, or up close and personal changes you've experienced.

Preparation for Day 7: Review the plan for Day 7, ensuring you're prepared for the next day's meals and activities. Consider how you can continue to broaden your detoxification tries and sponsorship your body's typical recovering cycles.

Day 6 Recap and Reflection

As you complete Day 6, you're most likely going to be more in accordance with your body's responses to the detox. It's essential to perceive the work your body is doing to sanitize and reestablish itself. The present fortified detoxification attempts are expected to utilize your body's energy, driving further into the cleaning framework while promising you stay supported and maintained.

CHAPTER 7

Day 7: Consolidating Detox Gains

On Day 7, you're entering the last period of the detox. This day is tied in with combining the additions you've made, zeroing in on supporting the advantages of the detox, and getting ready for a continuous change back to day to day existence, while keeping up with the sound propensities you've created.

Wake-up routine

Awaken Drink: Start your day with a relieving cup of warm water blended in with honey and cinnamon. This blend is known for its mitigating properties and can assist with settling glucose levels, giving a delicate beginning to your morning.

Care Practice: Burn through 15 minutes in quiet contemplation, considering your excursion up to this point. Center around the positive changes you've seen and set aims for how you need to keep integrating these detox standards into your life.

Breakfast

Buckwheat Flapjacks with New Berries: Get ready hotcakes utilizing buckwheat flour, a sans gluten elective that is wealthy in fiber and supplements. Top with new berries for a portion of cell reinforcements and a characteristic pleasantness.

Early in the day

Natural Lunch Break: Pick a tea that you've especially delighted in during the detox, whether for its flavor or how it affects you. Tasting gradually, relish this experience of harmony in your day.

Actual work: Practice Kendo or one more type of delicate hand to hand fighting for 20 minutes. This exercise advances equilibrium, quiet, and the progression of energy (Qi) all through the body, adjusting great to your detoxification endeavors.

Lunch

Blended Bean Salad in with Cilantro and Lime Dressing: Consolidate various beans (like kidney beans, dark beans, and chickpeas) with hacked cilantro, diced tomatoes, and avocado. Dress with lime juice and olive oil for a filling lunch that is high in fiber and protein.

Evening

Hydration Update: Proceed with your obligation to hydration. Maybe try different things with another mixture of natural products or spices to keep things fascinating and support your water's detoxifying power.

Careful Second: Designate time for a mobile reflection, in a perfect world some place you can interface with nature. Center around each step, every breath, and the magnificence around you, supporting an association with the current second.

Supper

Barbecued Vegetable Sticks with Quinoa Tabouleh: String zucchini, chime peppers, mushrooms, and onions on sticks, barbecue, and present with a side of quinoa tabouleh. This light yet nutritious dinner is loaded with nutrients, minerals, and fiber, supporting your body's continuous detoxification endeavors.

Evening Custom

Intelligent Journaling: Consider all the more profoundly your detox insight. What examples have you realized? How would you feel truly and inwardly? Start pondering how you can incorporate these bits of knowledge into your regular day to day existence.

Delicate Yoga: Take part in a 30-minute delicate yoga meeting, zeroing in on represents that advance unwinding and processing. This assists with merging the day's detox endeavors and set up your body for rest.

Groundwork for Day 8: Look forward to the last days of your detox. Begin arranging how you will keep on integrating the standards and practices you've learned into your customary daily schedule, guaranteeing a smooth progress and supported benefits.

Day 7 Recap and Reflection

Finishing Day 7 denotes a huge achievement in your detox process. At this point, you ought to begin feeling the significant impacts of your endeavors, from expanded energy and lucidity to worked on stomach related wellbeing and a more prominent feeling of prosperity. The present spotlight on uniting gains and considering your experience is essential for making this detox a groundbreaking and enduring change in your life.

CHAPTER 8

Day 8: Preparing for Transition

As you start Day 8, the center movements toward getting ready for the change out of the detox stage while holding the positive propensities you've created. This day is tied in with coordinating the standards of detoxification into a manageable, solid way of life.

Wake-up routine

Awaken Drink: Begin your day with a glass of warm water and a cut of natural lemon. This ceremonial guides processing and liver capability, and it's a sound propensity worth going on past the detox period.

Care Practice: Take part in a 10-minute directed representation zeroing in on your future, imagining yourself keeping up with these solid propensities and feeling lively, stimulated, and settled.

Breakfast

Vegetable Omelet with Avocado: Prepare an omelet with your number one vegetables, like spinach, tomatoes, and mushrooms. Present with cut avocado as an afterthought for a portion of sound fats and fiber. This protein-rich breakfast upholds supported energy levels and satiety.

Early in the day

Home grown Lunch Break: Settle on a natural tea that you've seen as especially gainful during the detox. Ponder how some tea has been a snapshot of delay and sustenance for your body.

Active work: Require a 20-minute energetic walk outside. Natural air and development are phenomenal for helping your temperament and flow.

Lunch

Soba Noodles with Edamame and Spring Vegetables: Set up a dish with soba noodles, edamame, and a variety of spring vegetables like asparagus and carrots, threw in a light sesame dressing. This feast offers a decent equilibrium of complex carbs, protein, and fundamental supplements.

Evening

Hydration Update: Keep up your hydration propensities, expecting to drink a lot of water over the course of the evening. Try different things with adding new natural product or home grown ice solid shapes for an invigorating turn.

Careful Second: Practice profound breathing or a short reflection to focus yourself, particularly on the off chance that you experience any stressors. Perceiving and overseeing pressure is significant for keeping up with equilibrium and wellbeing.

Supper

Simmered Chicken with Yam and Greens: Partake in a basic, feeding supper of cooked chicken, prepared yam, and a side of sautéed greens like kale or Swiss chard. This fair feast gives protein, complex starches, and an abundance of nutrients and minerals.

Evening Custom

Arranging Meeting: Get some margin to design your feasts and exercises for the next few days. Integrating detox standards into your customary routine can assist with supporting the advantages you've encountered.

Epsom Salt Shower: Enjoy a loosening up Epsom salt shower to calm muscles and advance a soothing night's rest. Adding a couple of drops of medicinal oil like lavender can upgrade the unwinding experience.

Groundwork for Day 9: Ponder the parts of the detox that you've seen as generally charming or advantageous, and contemplate how you can keep on applying these works on going ahead.

Day 8 Recap and Reflection

Day 8 is a urgent place where you start to look forward, arranging how to keep up with the positive changes you've made during the detox. It's tied in with perceiving the advantages of these solid propensities and tracking down ways of coordinating them into your regular routine for enduring wellbeing and essentialness.

CHAPTER 9

Day 8: Preparing for Transition

As you start Day 8, the center movements toward getting ready for the change out of the detox stage while holding the positive propensities you've created. This day is tied in with coordinating the standards of detoxification into a practical, sound way of life.

Wake-up routine

Awaken Drink: Begin your day with a glass of warm water and a cut of natural lemon. This ceremonial guides processing and liver capability, and it's a solid propensity worth going on past the detox period.

Care Practice: Take part in a 10-minute directed representation zeroing in on your future, imagining yourself keeping up with these solid propensities and feeling lively, stimulated, and settled.

Breakfast

Vegetable Omelet with Avocado: Prepare an omelet with your number one vegetables, like spinach, tomatoes, and mushrooms. Present with cut avocado as an afterthought for a portion of solid fats and fiber. This protein-rich breakfast upholds supported energy levels and satiety.

Early in the day

Natural Coffee Break: Choose a home grown tea that you've seen as especially gainful during the detox. Consider how some tea has been a snapshot of delay and sustenance for your body.

Active work: Require a 20-minute lively walk outside. Natural air and development are great for helping your state of mind and flow.

Lunch

Soba Noodles with Edamame and Spring Vegetables: Set up a dish with soba noodles, edamame, and a variety of spring vegetables like asparagus and carrots, threw in a light sesame dressing. This dinner offers a decent equilibrium of complex carbs, protein, and fundamental supplements.

Evening

Hydration Update: Keep up your hydration propensities, expecting to drink a lot of water over the course of the evening. Try different things with adding new natural product or home grown ice 3D shapes for a reviving turn.

Careful Second: Practice profound breathing or a short reflection to focus yourself, particularly on the off chance that you experience any stressors. Perceiving and overseeing pressure is urgent for keeping up with equilibrium and wellbeing.

Supper

Broiled Chicken with Yam and Greens: Partake in a straightforward, sustaining supper of simmered chicken, heated yam, and a side of sautéed greens like kale or Swiss chard. This fair dinner gives protein, complex starches, and an abundance of nutrients and minerals.

Evening Custom

Arranging Meeting: Get some margin to design your feasts and exercises for the next few days. Integrating detox standards into your normal routine can assist with supporting the advantages you've encountered.

Epsom Salt Shower: Enjoy a loosening up Epsom salt shower to calm muscles and advance a serene night's rest. Adding a couple of drops of natural ointment like lavender can upgrade the unwinding experience.

Groundwork for Day 9: Consider the parts of the detox that you've seen as generally charming or gainful, and contemplate how you can keep on applying these works on proceeding.

Day 8 Recap and Reflection

Day 8 is a crucial place where you start to look forward, arranging how to keep up with the positive changes you've made during the detox. It's tied in with perceiving the advantages of these sound propensities and tracking down ways of coordinating them into your day to day routine for enduring wellbeing and essentialness.

CHAPTER 10

Day 9: Embracing Long-Term Wellness

On Day 9, you're moving toward the completion of the detox program. This stage is connected to developing the inclinations you've created and examining how to embrace long stretch prosperity past the detox. This moment is the best opportunity to contemplate the movements you've experienced and to zero in on continuing with those practices that have been for the most part beneficial for your prosperity and success.

Awaken schedule

Stir Drink: Partake in some warm green tea around the start of today. Green tea is stacked with cell fortifications, maintains processing, and can be a remarkable extension to your morning plan for long stretch prosperity.

Care Practice: Commit 10 minutes to journaling, focusing in on appreciation. Record somewhere near three prosperity related pieces of your life that you're appreciative for. Practicing appreciation can overhaul your near and dear thriving and engage an elevating viewpoint on life.

Breakfast

Greek Yogurt with Granola and Mixed Berries: Participate in a bowl of Greek yogurt polished off with a high-fiber granola and different berries. This mix gives probiotics, protein, fiber, and cell fortifications, making it a fair, nutritious breakfast.

Promptly in the day

Regular Mid-day Break: Pick a calming local tea, similar to chamomile or lavender, to appreciate as a promptly in the dawn. These flavors can help with diminishing tension and advance loosening up, adding to in everyday flourishing.

Genuine work: Do a 20-minute stretching out daily schedule to additionally foster flexibility and stream. Common expanding can help with hindering injuries and advance a sensation of physical and mental balance.

Lunch

Grilled Chicken Plate of leafy greens with Mixed Greens and Vinaigrette: Accumulate a serving of leafy greens with grilled chicken chest, mixed greens, cherry tomatoes, cucumbers, and avocado, wearing a hand made olive oil and lemon vinaigrette. This supper is balanced with lean protein, sound fats, and different enhancements.

Evening

Hydration Update: Continue to zero in on hydration, investigating various roads with respect to various typical flavorings like mint leaves or slice normal item to keep it captivating and restoring.

Cautious Second: Take a short walk or find a quiet spot to practice care or significant unwinding for 5-10 minutes, focusing in on the ongoing second and the sensations in your body.

Dinner

Warmed Salmon with Quinoa and Steamed Broccoli: Set up a salmon filet ready with lemon and flavors, served nearby quinoa and steamed broccoli. This heart-great supper is rich in omega-3 unsaturated fats, protein, and fiber.

Evening Custom

Smart Planning: Contribute energy contemplating your post-detox targets and how you can incorporate the strong inclinations you've spread out into your everyday day to day practice. Organizing is basic to supporting these movements long stretch.

Loosening up Time: Make a section in a relaxing move you appreciate, such as scrutinizing a book, focusing on calming music, or practicing sensitive yoga. Loosening up is a huge piece of for the most part prosperity and can additionally foster rest quality.

Foundation for Day 10: Anticipate the last day of the detox program. Consider how you'll adulate your achievements and how you'll continue to execute these sound chips away at continuing.

Day 9 Recap and Reflection

Day 9 is connected to solidifying the commitment to long stretch wellbeing and considering how the guidelines of detox can be acclimated to your normal everyday presence. It's an opportunity to see the worth in the trip you've embraced and to expect a future where these newfound penchants become a trademark piece of your lifestyle.

CHAPTER 11

Day 10: Reflecting and Moving Forward

Great on appearing at Day 10 of your detox cycle! Today is about reflection and joy. It's everyday to see the value in all the irksome work you've placed into detoxifying your body and psyche and to spread out goals for going on with your excursion toward flourishing and prosperity.

Stir plan

Mix Drink: Start your day with an enabling glass of cucumber and mint-pervaded water. This drink is hydrating and assists with flushing hurts from your framework, tending to a new beginning and the fresh start you've pursued.

Care Practice: Participate in a 15-minute assessment zeroing in on recovery and positive suspicions. Think about your accomplishments and how you've made over these 10 days, characterizing your targets for how you wish to happen with the tendencies you've made.

Breakfast

Superfood Smoothie Bowl: Mix a blend of spinach, frozen berries, a banana, almond milk, and a scoop of protein powder. Top with cut ordinary things, nuts, and seeds for an upgrade pressed breakfast that is both delectable and empowering.

Immediately in the day

Nearby Speedy rest: Take part in some your super ordinary tea from the detox program, appreciating the taste and the see of quietness it brings.

Dynamic work: Require a pleasing 30-minute stroll around nature, zeroing in on the greatness around you and the vibe of prospering inside you. Strolling isn't just obviously appropriate for genuine flourishing yet additionally for mental clearness.

Lunch

Avocado and Chickpea Wrap: Fill an entire grain or sans gluten wrap with squashed avocado, cooked chickpeas, new veggies, and a sprinkle of tahini. This dinner is an ideal blend of sound fats, protein, and fiber.

Evening

Hydration Update: Keep a water bottle close by and keep on hydrating over the course of the evening. Keep in mind, hydration is essential to remaining mindful of the detoxification processes in your body.

Wary Second: Put forward essentially no energy in the early evening to unassumingly mull over your detox cycle. See the work you've caused and how it's affected you.

Supper

Barbecued Vegetable Platter with Quinoa Salad: Perceive your last day of the detox with a magnificent platter of barbecued vegetables, for example, cost peppers, zucchini, eggplant, and asparagus, served close by a quinoa salad blended in with flavors and lemon dressing. This supper is an eating experience for the assets and an appearance of the ideal, incredible counting calories tendencies you've made.

Evening Custom

Celebratory Reflection: Structure a letter to yourself, seeing your achievements and illustrating how you hope to keep on integrating the outlines learned into your ordinary everyday practice. Recognition your devotion and obligation to better thriving.

Relaxing: Permit yourself an opportunity to relax absolutely, maybe with a book or a delicate yoga meeting, embracing the quiet and satisfaction of finishing the detox program.

Establishment for Later: As you plan for life post-detox, consider the schedules and food groupings that have helped you most. Plan your feasting encounters and exercises for the going with a few days, guaranteeing a smooth change while remaining mindful of the center rules of your detox connection.

Day 10 Recap and Reflection

Finishing the 10-day detox is a gigantic accomplishment. It's about the authentic detoxification as well as about the psychological and very close recuperation you've encountered. As you push ahead, convey with you the thought, dietary affinities, and managing oneself practices you've made. These will go probably as your establishment for a went on with experience towards success and flourishing.

CHAPTER 12

Recipes and Meal Plans

Making a thorough assortment of recipes and feast plans for a 10-day detox includes offering an assortment of nutritious, clean, and detox-accommodating choices. These recipes are intended to help the body's regular detoxification processes while giving pleasant and fulfilling dinners. Here, I'll frame a determination of recipes for breakfast, lunch, supper, and tidbits that can be blended and matched throughout the detox. Furthermore, I'll give an example 3-day feast plan that can be adjusted or rehashed all through the detox period.

Detox Recipes

Breakfast Options

1. Green Detox Smoothie:
     ◦ 1 cup spinach leaves
     ◦ 1/2 avocado
     ◦ 1/2 banana
     ◦ 1/2 cup frozen pineapple chunks
     ◦ 1 tablespoon chia seeds
     ◦ 1 cup unsweetened almond milk
     ◦ Blend all ingredients until smooth.
2. Oatmeal with Berries and Nuts:
     ◦ 1/2 cup rolled oats, cooked in water

- ◦ 1/2 cup mixed berries (blueberries, raspberries)
- ◦ A sprinkle of almonds and walnuts
- ◦ A dash of cinnamon
- ◦ Combine cooked oatmeal with toppings.

Lunch Options

1. Quinoa Salad with Roasted Vegetables:
   - ◦ 1/2 cup cooked quinoa
   - ◦ 1 cup mixed roasted vegetables (bell peppers, zucchini, broccoli)
   - ◦ 1 tablespoon olive oil
   - ◦ 1 tablespoon lemon juice
   - ◦ Salt and pepper to taste
   - ◦ Toss quinoa and vegetables with dressing ingredients.
2. Detox Veggie Soup:
   - ◦ 1 tablespoon olive oil
   - ◦ 1 onion, chopped
   - ◦ 2 garlic cloves, minced
   - ◦ 2 carrots, diced
   - ◦ 2 celery stalks, diced
   - ◦ 1 cup chopped kale
   - ◦ 4 cups vegetable broth
   - ◦ 1 can diced tomatoes
   - ◦ Herbs (thyme, oregano)
   - ◦ Salt and pepper to taste
   - ◦ Sauté onion and garlic, add vegetables and broth, simmer until veggies are tender.

Dinner Options

1. Baked Salmon with Steamed Broccoli:
   - ◦ 1 salmon fillet
   - ◦ 1 tablespoon olive oil

- ◦ 1 teaspoon lemon zest
- ◦ 2 cups broccoli, steamed
- ◦ Season salmon with olive oil, lemon zest, salt, and pepper. Bake at 375°F for 12-15 minutes. Serve with steamed broccoli.

2. Stir-Fried Tofu with Mixed Greens:
   - ◦ 1 block firm tofu, cubed
   - ◦ 1 tablespoon coconut oil
   - ◦ 2 cups mixed greens (spinach, kale)
   - ◦ 2 tablespoons tamari sauce
   - ◦ 1 garlic clove, minced
   - ◦ Stir-fry tofu in coconut oil until golden, add greens and garlic, cook until wilted, add tamari sauce.

Snack Options

1. Cucumber and Hummus:
   - ◦ Sliced cucumber
   - ◦ 1/4 cup hummus
   - ◦ Enjoy cucumber slices dipped in hummus.
2. Fruit and Nut Mix:
   - ◦ 1/4 cup mixed unsalted nuts (almonds, walnuts)
   - ◦ 1/4 cup dried fruits (apricots, figs)
   - ◦ Combine nuts and dried fruits for a quick snack.

3-Day Detox Meal Plan
Day 1

- Breakfast: Green Detox Smoothie
- Mid-Morning Snack: Apple slices with almond butter
- Lunch: Quinoa Salad with Roasted Vegetables
- Afternoon Snack: Cucumber and Hummus
- Dinner: Baked Salmon with Steamed Broccoli

Day 2

- Breakfast: Oatmeal with Berries and Nuts
- Mid-Morning Snack: Fruit and Nut Mix
- Lunch: Detox Veggie Soup
- Afternoon Snack: A green apple
- Dinner: Stir-Fried Tofu with Mixed Greens

Day 3

- Breakfast: Green Detox Smoothie
- Mid-Morning Snack: Carrot sticks with hummus
- Lunch: Quinoa Salad with Avocado and Black Beans
    - Follow the Quinoa Salad recipe, adding 1/2 an avocado (diced) and 1/4 cup rinsed black beans
- Afternoon Snack: A handful of almonds
- Dinner: Grilled Chicken or Portobello Mushrooms with a side of Roasted Sweet Potatoes
    - Season chicken or mushrooms with herbs and olive oil, grill until cooked. Serve with roasted sweet potatoes seasoned with cinnamon.

This 3-day feast plan offers a fair way to deal with a detox diet, with an accentuation on entire food sources, lean proteins, and a lot of products of the soil. These feasts are intended to help the body's detoxification cycle while guaranteeing you stay fed and fulfilled. Go ahead and change bits and fixings as indicated by your own inclinations and dietary necessities.

CHAPTER 13

Maintaining Benefits Post-Detox

Progressing out of the 10-day detox doesn't spell almost certain doom for the excursion; rather, it's the start of coordinating better propensities into your everyday existence. Keeping up with the advantages post-detox includes going on with careful eating, remaining hydrated, consolidating actual work, and rehearsing pressure the executives. This stage is critical for long haul achievement and guaranteeing the positive changes become a super durable piece of your way of life.

Embracing Another Typical

Careful Eating: One of the main examples from the detox is the significance of being aware of what you eat. Pay attention to your body's appetite and completion signals, pick entire food varieties over handled choices, and appreciate each nibble. This approach can change your relationship with food, prompting enduring medical advantages.

Hydration: Proceeding to drink a lot of water is fundamental. Hydration supports processing, keeps up with energy levels, and supports by and large physical processes. Regularly practice it to begin your day with a glass of water and keep a water bottle helpful over the course of the day.

Adjusted Diet: Consolidate different organic products, vegetables, entire grains, lean proteins, and sound fats into your feasts. A decent eating regimen guarantees you're getting many supplements fundamental for keeping up with energy, insusceptibility, and by and large wellbeing.

Supporting Detox Advantages

Ordinary Detox Practices: Integrate components of the detox into your normal daily schedule. This could mean beginning every day with a detoxifying drink, as warm lemon water, or carving out opportunity every week for taking care of oneself practices that assist with overseeing pressure and detoxify the body, like yoga or sauna meetings.

Limit Poison Openness: Keep on limiting openness to poisons by picking natural food varieties while conceivable, utilizing normal cleaning and individual consideration items, and staying away from ecological poisons like tobacco smoke and contamination.

Stomach Wellbeing: The detox probably worked on your stomach related wellbeing, so keep it a need. Incorporate probiotic and prebiotic-rich food sources in your eating regimen to help a sound stomach microbiome, which is essential for processing, resistance, and even state of mind guideline.

Actual work and Stress The executives

Customary Activity: Find proactive tasks you appreciate and make them a piece of your daily practice. Practice not just aides in overseeing weight and diminishing the gamble of persistent sicknesses yet in addition helps your mind-set and energy levels.

Stress Decrease: Go on with care practices like reflection, profound breathing activities, or journaling. Overseeing pressure is indispensable for forestalling the development of poisons and keeping up with mental clearness and close to home equilibrium.

Long haul Obligation to Wellbeing

Persistent Learning: Remain informed about sustenance, exercise, and wellbeing to come to taught conclusions about your wellbeing. The excursion doesn't end following 10 days; it's a constant course of learning and adjusting.

Local area Backing: Encircle yourself with a local area that upholds your wellbeing objectives. This could be companions, family, or online networks. Sharing encounters and difficulties can give inspiration and responsibility.

Change and Customize: As you push ahead, recall that what works for one individual may not work for another. Pay attention to your body, and change your propensities and schedules to meet your remarkable necessities and objectives.

Incorporation into Day to day existence

As you reintegrate into your ordinary routine post-detox, the key is to bring the examples learned and the propensities shaped during the detox into your day to day existence. This doesn't mean you want to live as prohibitively as you did during the detox, but instead that you embrace a more cognizant and wellbeing centered way to deal with living.

The finish of the 10-day detox is only the start of a better, more careful approach to everyday life. By proceeding to apply the standards picked up during the detox, you can keep up with the advantages long haul and partake in a more excellent of life. The progress might require tolerance and tirelessness, yet the compensations of supported wellbeing, energy, and prosperity are certainly worth the work. Embrace this new ordinary with certainty, realizing you have the apparatuses and information to help your wellbeing and joy.

Conclusion

As we arrive at the finish of "The 10-Day Detox: Purge Your Body, Clear Your Brain," now is the right time to consider the excursion we've set out upon together. This detox was not just about the brief end of poisons from our bodies; it was tied in with starting an extraordinary excursion towards better wellbeing, expanded energy, and more prominent mental lucidity. As you stand at this crossroads, you have the information, instruments, and encounters to keep encouraging a way of life that upholds your general prosperity.

The Excursion of Change

Throughout recent days, you've found a way huge ways to lessen your poison load, feed your body with energizing food sources, participate in actual work, and practice care to clear your psyche. You've probably experienced difficulties en route, however you've additionally found new qualities and bits of knowledge about your wellbeing and propensities. This course of detoxification has not exclusively been tied in with purifying your actual body yet additionally about shedding propensities that never again serve you, making space for new, wellbeing supporting practices.

Supported Wellbeing and Prosperity

The finish of this detox doesn't imply the finish of your wellbeing process; rather, it's a fresh start. The practices you've taken on and the information you've acquired structure a strong groundwork whereupon you can fabricate a supported, solid way of life. Keep in mind, the way to keeping up with the advantages of this detox is consistency and care in your decisions.

•Careful Eating: Keep on picking entire, supplement thick food varieties that help your body's regular detoxification processes. Pay attention to your body's yearning and completion signals, and eat with expectation and appreciation.

•Standard Actual work: Integrate actual work that you appreciate into your day to day everyday practice. Whether it's yoga, strolling, cycling, or one more type of activity, normal development upholds your body's wellbeing and upgrades your mind-set.

•Continuous Care Practice: Keep care rehearses a piece of your everyday existence, whether through contemplation, journaling, or basically taking minutes to inhale and be available. These practices lessen pressure and work on mental clearness.

•Hydration: Keep on focusing on hydration, holding back nothing 8 glasses of water a day. Hydration is critical to supporting detoxification and generally speaking wellbeing.

Embracing Difficulties and Observing Triumphs

As you push ahead, you'll unavoidably confront difficulties and impediments. Keep in mind, each challenge is a chance for development and learning. Remain adaptable, change your practices on a case by case basis, and be caring to yourself through the promising and less promising times. Praise your triumphs, regardless of how little, and perceive the headway you've made.

A Deep rooted Excursion

Your wellbeing and prosperity are a deep rooted venture, not an objective. The "10-Day Detox" is a venturing stone towards a better, more energetic life. Keep on investigating, learn, and adjust your propensities to help your wellbeing objectives. Remain inquisitive about your body's necessities, and be available to attempting new food sources, exercises, and care rehearses.

All in all

Congrats on finishing the "10-Day Detox: Purge Your Body, Clear Your Psyche." You've made a significant stride towards improving your wellbeing and prosperity. As you forge ahead with your excursion, recall that the decisions every day are strong determinants of your wellbeing and satisfaction. Utilize the information and propensities you've developed during this detox as an establishment for a deep rooted obligation to prosperity.

Much thanks to you for permitting this book to be a piece of your wellbeing process. May you push ahead with certainty, engaged by the information that you have the apparatuses and solidarity to help your body and brain. Here's to a better, more joyful you.